K.-J. Zülch

Die geschichtliche Entwicklung der deutschen Neurologie

Historical Development of German Neurology

Mit 10 Abbildungen

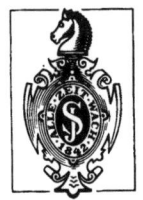

Springer-Verlag
Berlin Heidelberg New York
London Paris Tokyo

Professor Dr. Dr. h.c. KLAUS-JOACHIM ZÜLCH
Emer. Direktor am Max-Planck-Institut f. Hirnforschung
und der
Neurol. Klinik des Städt. Krankenhauses Köln-Merheim
Ostmerheimer-Straße 200
5000 Köln 91

ISBN 978-3-642-52287-1   ISBN 978-3-642-71903-5 (eBook)
DOI 10.1007/978-3-642-71903-5

CIP-Kurztitelaufnahme der Deutschen Bibliothek. Zülch, Klaus-J.: Die geschichtliche Entwicklung der deutschen Neurologie = Historical development of German neurology / K.-J. Zülch. – Berlin ; Heidelberg ; New York ; London ; Paris ; Tokyo : Springer, 1987.

Dieses Werk ist urheberrechtlich geschützt. Die dadurch begründeten Rechte, insbesondere die der Übersetzung, des Nachdrucks, des Vortrags, der Entnahme von Abbildungen und Tabellen, der Funksendung, der Mikroverfilmung oder der Vervielfältigung auf anderen Wegen und der Speicherung in Datenverarbeitungsanlagen, bleiben, auch bei nur auszugsweiser Verwertung, vorbehalten. Eine Vervielfältigung dieses Werkes oder von Teilen dieses Werkes ist auch im Einzelfall nur in den Grenzen der gesetzlichen Bestimmungen des Urheberrechtsgesetzes der Bundesrepublik Deutschland vom 9. September 1965 in der Fassung vom 24. Juni 1985 zulässig. Sie ist grundsätzlich vergütungspflichtig. Zuwiderhandlungen unterliegen den Strafbestimmungen des Urheberrechtsgesetzes.

© Springer-Verlag Berlin Heidelberg 1987

Die geschichtliche Entwicklung der deutschen Neurologie

Ansprache zur Eröffnung des Weltkongresses für Neurologie in Hamburg, 1985

Herr Regierender Bürgermeister, meine Herren Präsidenten und Sekretäre, verehrte Damen und Herren!

Wir freuen uns, daß Sie, die Neurologen der Welt, zum erstenmal in der Geschichte der Neurologie zu Ihrem Weltkongreß 1985 zu uns nach Deutschland gekommen sind. Das ist eine besondere Ehre auch für Hamburg, die Wirkungsstätte von Max Nonne (1861–1959), einem der großen Neurologen dieses Landes, der hier im alten Eppendorfer Krankenhaus von 1884 bereits im Jahre 1896 die erste neurologische Abteilung aufbaute. Er erhielt 1919 bei der Gründung der Universität den ersten neurologischen Lehrstuhl unseres Landes.

Zur Einstimmung auf diesen Kongreß möchte ich Sie mit der geschichtlichen Entwicklung der deutschen Neurologie bekanntmachen. Dazu beschreibe ich zunächst das allgemeine Bild der Neurologie an der Wende vom 18. zum 19. Jahrhundert und nenne dazu einige prominente neurologisch arbeitende Ärzte dieser Zeit. Damals erhielt die Medizin in Europa ihre naturwissenschaftliche Begründung.

Anfänge der Neurologie

Erinnern wir uns: Lange zuvor war schon durch Thomas Willis (1622–1675) der Begriff der „Neurologie" geschaffen worden, als er neben die „Osteologia" und „Myologia" eine „Neurologia" als selbständige Disziplin stellte.

Welche Akzente setzte nun diese neue Wissenschaft der Neurologie ein Jahrhundert später? Damals hatte Marshall Hall (1790–1875) seine Reflextheorie entwickelt, James Parkinson (1755–1824) die Schüttellähmung als einheitliches Krankheitsbild beschrieben und Charles Bell (1747–1842) die Funktion der spinalen Wurzeln erfaßt. Weiter war es François Magendie (1783–1855) gelungen, die Vorgänge im Rückenmark aufzuklären und Jean Cruveilhier (1791–1874) hatte seinen großartigen Atlas der pathologischen Anatomie des Nervensystems veröffentlicht. In Italien hatte Giovanni Battista Morgagni (1682–1771) für alle Gebiete die ersten pathologischen Grundlagen der Krankheiten beschrieben (z. B. der Apoplexie) und Luigi Galvani (1737–1798) gezeigt, daß bei der Muskeltätigkeit elektrische Ströme entstehen können. Der so vielseitig begabte genialische Alexander von Humboldt (1769–1859) konnte diese Erkenntnisse bei seinen experimentellen Arbeiten nutzen. Diese führten zur Begründung einer Nervenphysiologie. Sonst aber waren in Deutschland in dieser Zeit nur Johann Christian Reil (1759–1843) mit seinen ersten Vorstellungen über das Zusammenwirken der Hirnteile zu einem Ganzen bekannt geworden. Schließlich hatte Samuel Thomas Soemmering (1755–1830) das Hirn als das Organ der Seele herausgestellt; auch hatte er erstmalig die Hirnnerven richtig eingeteilt.

Aufbruch in Berlin: Die Gründung der Universität

Dieses sind einige der wichtigsten wissenschaftlichen Ergebnisse, die Mosaikhaft die damaligen Kenntnisse der Funktionen des Nervensystems zeichnen. Vor diesem Hintergrund tritt nun aber in Berlin im ersten Drittel des 19. Jahrhunderts plötzlich eine Generation junger

Forscher auf die Bühne der Wissenschaft, angeregt offenbar besonders durch einen Anatomen, der dann aber auch zum Physiologen wurde: Johannes Müller (1801–1858) (Abb. 1), ein Schüler des Physiologen Asmund Rudolphi.

Müller war bereits mit 31 Jahren auf den Lehrstuhl nach Berlin gerufen worden. Er beendete die Begründung der Medizin auf die „Naturphilosophie". Bereits wenige Jahre später konnte er sein großes „Handbuch der Physiologie" veröffentlichen, das ein faszinierendes Bild der nervalen Funktionen bei Mensch und Tier zeichnete.

Von seinen direkten Schülern seien hier nur folgende Namen genannt: Theodor Schwann (1810–1862), der bald nach Belgien auf den Lehrstuhl in Löwen berufen wurde, Friedrich Gustav Jakob Henle (1809–1885), der in die Schweiz auf den Züricher Lehrstuhl ging, Heinrich Friedrich Bidder (1810–1884), der an die deutsche Universität von Dorpat zurückkehrte, und schließlich auch Robert Remak (1815–1865), der in Berlin eine ganze Generation von Anatomen ausbildete. Die Zahl der Schüler und Mitarbeiter von Johannes Müller war aber weit größer. Nennen wir die Physiologen DuBois-Reymond (1818–1896), Carl Ludwig (1816–1895) und Ernst Brücke (1819–1892). Nennen wir weiter die Anatomen Albert Koelliker (1817–1905), Friedrich Leopold Goltz (1834–1902) und den genialen Hermann von Helmholtz (1821–1894), den Erfinder des Augenspiegels, um dessen Zugehörigkeit sich später Ophthalmologen, Physiologen und Anatomen gleichermaßen gestritten haben. Selbst Rudolf Virchow, der Pathologe (1821–1902), und der Chirurg Theodor Billroth (1829–1894) – später Privatdozent in Berlin und danach auf den Lehrstuhl in Wien berufen – wie auch der in der Diskussion um Darwin bekannte Naturwissenschaftler Ernst Haeckel (1824–1912), haben sich selbst als Schüler von Johannes Müller bezeichnet. Schließlich gehörte auch der bereits als Privatdozent nach Graz berufene Otto Loewy zu denjenigen Wissenschaftlern, die bei Johannes Müller ihre ersten Schritte machten.

Man kann nur mit Staunen dieses explosive und aufsehenerregende Wachstum der Berliner Medizinischen Schule sehen, die, nach einem für Deutschland in der Medizin fast „leeren" 18. Jahrhundert, in so kurzer Zeit so viele weltberühmte Wissenschaftler hervorbringen konnte. Wahrscheinlich kann man dies nur aus der Zeit verstehen, die ich deshalb mit einigen Strichen zeichnen muß.

Europa war gerade von der Napoleonischen Herrschaft befreit worden. Der Aufbruch in Preußen wurde eingeleitet durch die Reden von Fichte und Schleiermacher in Berlin, die die Jugend geistig zum Kampf für die Freiheit Europas zu begeistern verstanden hatten. Zu diesen trat Wilhelm von Humboldt (1809) als Leiter des Unterrichtswesens, der seinem König ein neues Modell einer Universität entworfen hatte, in dem die Professoren frei von staatlicher Beeinflussung, sich der Forschung *und* der Lehre „gleichermaßen" widmen sollten. Auch schuf er als Vorbereitung einer solchen Universität das Gymnasium als die höhere Erziehungsschule. Der König folgte der Empfehlung zur Universitäts-Gründung in Berlin und betonte 1811: „Man müsse jetzt durch geistige Kräfte ersetzen, was an physischen verlorengegangen sei." In Preußen herrschte Hochstimmung für den Kampf gegen das napoleonische Regime und für eine freie Demokratie.

Doch wurde in der Folge die Jugend in Europa durch die „Reaktion", die nach dem Wiener Kongreß die mitteleuropäischen Staaten beherrschte, um ihre demokratischen Freiheitsideale betrogen. Vergeblich war, daß so mancher ihrer neuen akademischen Lehrer gemeinsam mit den Studenten auf den Straßen und den Barrikaden dafür gekämpft hatte.

Mag sein, daß sich diese politische Begeisterung zum Studium an den Universitäten sublimierte, jedenfalls blühte dieses Modell der neuen Universität in Berlin auf und brachte erstaunliche Erfolge in der Wissenschaft.

Aber auch in der Folge blieb die Unterdrückung der erhofften Freiheit bestehen und führte immer wieder zu den bekannten politischen Erhebungen der Jahre 1832 und 1848.

Moritz-Heinrich Romberg, der erste neurologische Kliniker

Für die Neurologie aber gibt es jetzt ein neues Phänomen: die Person des jungen Internisten Moritz-Heinrich Romberg (1786–1873) (Abb. 2). Er wird 1840 zum Direktor des Königlich-Poliklinischen Institutes in Berlin ernannt. Es ist überaus erstaunlich, daß er bereits im gleichen Jahr mit der Veröffentlichung seiner klinischen Erfahrungen im ersten Band seines „Lehrbuches der Nervenkrankheiten des Menschen" beginnen konnte. Das Buch wird rasch ins Englische übersetzt und bereits nach kurzer Zeit übt es seinen Einfluß auch in England und Amerika aus. Wie hoch Kalinowski und Houston Merrit/USA in unserer Zeit die Bedeutung dieses jungen Neurologen werten, zeigt, daß sie die Errichtung der Rombergschen Klinik als den „Beginn der Neurologie" überhaupt bezeichnen. Auch Ramsay Hunt (USA) nennt Rombergs Lehrbuch die „erste systematische Beschreibung der Neurologie" in der inneren Klinik (1933/34).

Offensichtlich wirkt diese erste zündende Veröffentlichung in dem neuen Fach befruchtend auf das übrige Deutschland, wo wir jetzt die großen Kliniker dieser Jahrzehnte sich entwickeln sehen, wie Nikolaus Friedreich (1825–1882) in Würzburg und Heidelberg (Abb. 3), Adolf Kussmaul (1822–1902) in Erlangen, Ernst Leyden (1832–1919) in Berlin, Adolf Strümpell (1856–1925) in Leipzig (Abb. 4), Friedrich Schultze (1845–1935) in Göttingen, Paul Julius Möbius (1853–1907) in Leipzig, Ludwig Traube (1818–1876) in Berlin und Heinrich Curschmann d. Ä. (1846–1910) in Hamburg und Leipzig.

Beiträge der Grundlagenwissenschaften für die Neurologie

Aber der Funke springt auch auf die übrigen neurologischen Grundlagenfächer über und erzeugt einen neuen Enthusiasmus zur wissenschaftlichen Arbeit, die jetzt von der *Allgemeinpathologie* ausgeht. Ich nenne Friedrich Daniel von Recklinghausen (1833–1910), Julius Friedrich Cohnheim (1839–1884), Carl Weigert (1845–1904) und den großen Rudolf Virchow (1821–1902), der eine neue, durch den

Pathologen kontrollierte und jetzt pathogenetisch orientierte Klinik weltweit für dies Jahrhundert als Vorbild setzt.

Vertreter der *normalen Anatomie* und *Physiologie* schließen sich diesem Vorwärtsdrängen an: Albert Koelliker (1817–1905), Wilhelm His (1831–1904), Michael von Lenhossék in Würzburg (1863–1937) und Johann Purkinje (1787–1869) in Breslau sind würdige Vertreter ihrer Fächer. Der letzte wurde von der Karls-Universität in Prag als junger Prosektor nach Breslau berufen; er entwickelte dort das erste – von seinem Vorgänger gegründete – moderne physiologische Institut der Welt.

Wir sehen: jetzt drängen auch aus den Nachbarländern die jungen begabten Wissenschaftler zu den deutschen Universitäten, weil sie dort eine anregende geistige Sphäre und vorzügliche Arbeitsbedingungen vorfanden.

Die weitere Entwicklung in Berlin

So verlief das 19. Jahrhundert in Berlin und im übrigen Deutschland. Was aber folgte dem so überaus glücklichen Start der Neurologie unter Moritz Romberg in der Zeit des Wechsels zum 20. Jahrhundert? Gelang es jetzt nachzuholen, was bei den britischen Nachbarn in London mit dem National Hospital Queen Square und seinen großen Vertretern Victor Horsley, C. E. Beevor, Marcus Gunn, Charlton Bastian, Hughlings Jackson, W. R. Gowers und David Ferrier und schließlich Charles E. Brown-Sèquard sowie in Frankreich mit der Salpetrière und seinen Charcot, Broca, Dejerine, Babinski, und später Pierre Marie gelungen war, nämlich sich in der Hauptstadt ein zentrales Spitzeninstitut für Neurologie zu schaffen? Nein, das gelang nicht! Es war enttäuschend, was sich in der Neurologie in Berlin abspielte.

Zwar wurde als Nachfolger Rombergs der vorzügliche Wilhelm Griesinger (1817–1868) berufen; dieser hatte sich aber als Psychiater ein großes Programm zur Modernisierung und Humanisierung der Psychiatrie vorgenommen. Er erhielt auch in Berlin zu dem Romberg'schen Poliklinischen Institut – das weitgehend neurologisch ausgerichtet war – eine eigene psychiatrische Abteilung in der Charité. Die Masse der Neurologie aber ging mit der inneren Medizin in die Hände von Ernst von Leyden (1832–1910) über. Griesinger ist leider nicht mehr dazu gekommen, sein humanitäres Programm in Berlin voll zu verwirklichen, er starb früh und als Nachfolger wurde für seine Klinik Karl Westphal (1833–1890), ein Schüler Romberg's berufen. Aber auch Westphal wurde vorzeitig unheilbar krank und deshalb mußte bis zu seinem Tode, sein Lieblingsschüler Hermann Oppenheim (1858–1919) als kommissarischer Leiter eingesetzt werden.

Die Fakultät schlug dann auch Oppenheim unico loco als Nachfolger vor, doch wurde er vom Ministerium wegen seines Glaubens nicht berufen. Sicher hat Oppenheim Grund gehabt, tief gekränkt zu sein, war er doch der erste Typus eines reinen Neurologen gewesen und als solcher bereits bekannt in der ganzen Welt. Er mußte sich jetzt von der Universität zurückziehen und unterhielt eine private Poliklinik und ein Laboratorium aus eigenen Geldmitteln, blieb aber weiterhin persönlich so berühmt, daß zu ihm neurologische Patienten aus aller Welt strömten.

Schon 1896 konnte Hermann Oppenheim sein erschöpfend geschriebenes Lehrbuch der Neurologie veröffentlichen, das ihn sofort weithin bekannt machte. 7 deutsche Auflagen sowie 3 englische und je eine russische, spanische und italienische Übersetzung folgten. Er wurde tatsächlich zum „Praeceptor mundi" in der Neurologie, wie man damals sagte. Trotzdem: Oppenheim konnte nicht verwinden, daß er der Universität hatte den Rücken kehren müssen. Damit war eine „Sternstunde" für die Weiterentwicklung der Neurologie in Deutschland verpaßt, denn er, der bekannteste deutsche Neurologe, war ja nicht an die zentrale Schaltstätte nach Berlin gekommen.

Noch einmal hat sich später eine zweite gute Gelegenheit für die Entwicklung der Neurologie in Berlin und in Deutschland ergeben: Der Psychiater Emil Kraepelin (1856–1926) wurde 1912 von München auf den freigewordenen Berliner Lehrstuhl berufen. Kraepelin war weithin bekannt durch sein Lehrbuch mit einer ersten nosologischen Einteilung der psychiatrischen Krankheiten. Er stellte aber als

Berufungsbedingung für die Berliner Kanzel, daß gleichzeitig die Neurologie abgetrennt und als eigener Lehrstuhl mit Klinik, d. h. gesondert geführt werden sollte. Das aber wurde vom Berliner Ministerium abgelehnt.

Statt dessen wurde Karl Bonhoeffer (1868–1948) aus Breslau berufen, der wie sein Lehrer Wernicke, als der Prototyp eines Verfechters der „Neuropsychiatrie" angesehen werden muß. Auch für Bonhoeffer waren Geisteskrankheiten „Gehirnkrankheiten", wie für Griesinger und Karl Wernicke (1848–1905). Sie waren die ersten klar gezeichneten Führer einer Neuropsychiatrie, wie sie später in Deutschland durch Hoche, Bumke, Karl Kleist, Binswanger und Berger vertreten wurde. An den Universitäten blieb jetzt – mit wenigen Ausnahmen – die Neurologie in den Händen dieser Neuropsychiater.

Wäre damals ein eigener Lehrstuhl für Neurologie in Berlin geschaffen worden, so hätte das richtunggebend für die Entwicklung der deutschen Neurologie sein können. Das aber geschah nicht. Jetzt war die zweite und letzte „Sternstunde" der deutschen Neurologie vorübergegangen. Über die spätere katastrophale Entwicklung nach 1933, werden wir noch berichten.

Neurologie in der Inneren Medizin

Inzwischen müssen wir nachholen, was mit der Neurologie im Rahmen der inneren Medizin geschehen war. Was wurde aus dieser Wurzel? Der Internist Wilhelm Erb (1840–1921) in Heidelberg (Abb. 5), neurologisch außerordentlich interessiert und ein hervorragender Kenner der Muskelkrankheiten und der Elektrotherapie und -pathologie, war dort die entscheidende Persönlichkeit. Er hatte für sich als Professor der Inneren Medizin eine klare Entscheidung getroffen: „das Fach der ‚Nervenpathologie' – wie er damals die Neurologie nannte – sei zu breit, so schrieb er, als daß es noch gemeinsam mit der inneren Medizin von *einem* Wissenschaftler vertreten werden könne."

Erb betonte in einer großen Rede (1880), „daß es wohl keiner ausführlichen Darlegung mehr bedürfe, daß die eigentliche wissenschaftliche und mögliche fruchtbringende Bearbeitung der Nervenpathologie, heutzutage nur noch eine spezialistische sein könne: die ganze Hingabe, die ganze Arbeitskraft eines Mannes sei erforderlich, um dieses gewaltige Gebiet auch nur einigermaßen zu beherrschen, wie viel mehr um es selbständig und fruchtbringend zu bearbeiten...". Diese Einstellung hat er immer wieder über Jahrzehnte auf Kongressen betont.

Tatsächlich hat auch die deutsche Neurologie als Folge einer solchen Auffassung – im Gegensatz zu vielen anderen Ländern – später viel weniger Mühe gehabt, sich von der inneren Medizin zu trennen.

Neurologie an allgemeinen Krankenhäusern

Wie aber ging es dann mit der Neurologie weiter? Merkwürdigerweise kam eine große Unterstützung für das Fach aus dem Wirken bedeutender Persönlichkeiten an den Städtischen Großkrankenhäusern. Diese Hilfe ist nicht zu gering anzusetzen für die Entwicklung der deutschen Neurologie. So gelang es in Hannover (Ludwig Bruns, 1858–1916), in Dortmund (zeitweilig), Danzig (Adolf Wallenberg, 1862–1939) und in Breslau (Ludwig Mann, 1866–1936, neben Otfrid Foerster, (1873–1941) Städtische Abteilungen einzurichten.

Oben erwähnte ich schon die Tätigkeit von Max Nonne (1861–1959) in Hamburg (Abb. 6), der bereits 1896 am Allgemeinen Krankenhaus Eppendorf, eine eigene neurologische Klinik schuf. Max Nonne erreichte es in Hamburg, daß an allen Großkrankenhäusern eigene neurologische Abteilungen unter seinen Schülern eingerichtet wurden. Damit ist in Westdeutschland die klinische Neurologie in Hamburg wahrscheinlich am dichtesten vertreten.

Weiter sei hier besonders auf die neurologische Tätigkeit von Otfrid Foerster hingewiesen, dem es gelang, zu der neurologischen Klinik in einem Städtischen Krankenhaus, eine Sonderabteilung für Hirnverletzte einzurichten und schließlich sogar ein später weltbekanntes „Neurologisches Forschungsinstitut" aufzubauen.

Die großen neurologischen Forschungsinstitute

Otfrid Foerster (1873–1941) in Breslau (Abb. 7), war wohl der bedeutenste Neurologe, den Deutschland hervorgebracht hat. Er genoß großes Ansehen auch bei den Neurochirurgen. Die meisten amerikanischen Neurochirurgen der jetzt emeritierten älteren Generation, haben einige Zeit am neurologischen Forschungsinstitut in Breslau bei Otfrid Foerster verbracht, unter ihnen besonders Percival Bailey, Paul Bucy, Wilder Penfield und Josef P. Evans. Lange Zeit hat sich Otfrid Foerster die Mittel für seine Arbeitsstätte aus persönlichen Einkünften beschaffen müssen. Erst 1932 baute dann die Rockefeller-Stiftung – auf Empfehlung amerikanischer Freunde – zusammen mit dem Staat Preußen und der Stadt Breslau, das moderne Neurologische Forschungsinstitut. Aber damals war es eigentlich schon zu spät, der größte Teil des Lebenswerkes Otfrid Foerster war vollbracht. Dieses erhielt unter seinem Nachfolger in Breslau Viktor von Weizsäcker (Abb. 8) (1886–1957) den Namen „Otfrid Foerster-Institut".

Als zweite bedeutende Persönlichkeit im Kreis der Grundlagenforscher und neurologischen Kliniker, müssen wir Oskar Vogt (1876–1959) nennen, der mit seiner Frau Cécile das große Kaiser-Wilhelm-Institut in Berlin-Buch (Abb. 9) geschaffen hat. Auch er hat viele Jahrzehnte auf diesen Neubau warten müssen, hatte doch auch er mit einem kleinen Laboratorium – geschaffen aus eigenen Mitteln – anfangen müssen. Aus dem berühmten Berliner Institut sind hervorgegangen: Korbinian Brodmann (1868–1918) und Max Bielschowsky (1869–1940) sowie Timofjejew, der Genetiker; später hat Hugo Spatz (1888–1969) die Leitung übernommen und Julius Hallervorden (1882–1965) und Wilhelm Tönnis (1898–1978), als hervorragende Mitarbeiter gewonnen. Aber auch hier, wie in Breslau bei Otfrid Foerster und in München bei Emil Kraepelin – an der Forschungsanstalt für Psychiatrie – war es erst die Rockefeller-Stiftung, die durch großherzige Hilfe die Errichtung einer Großforschung in Berlin-Buch ermöglichte.

Die drei Institute sind eine bemerkenswerte Stütze für die Entwicklung der neurologischen Wissenschaften im deutschen

Sprachraum geworden, zudem ein Mekka in der Ausbildung für viele junge Wissenschaftler in der Welt. Breslau und Berlin-Buch gingen allerdings der Neurologie durch den letzten Krieg verloren.

Die Neuropathologen

Wir erwähnten die in Berlin-Buch tätigen Neuropathologen und müssen jetzt als Mitarbeiter des Münchener Kaiser-Wilhelm-Institutes für Psychiatrie unter Emil Kraepelin (1856–1926) besonders herausstellen: Franz Nissl (1860–1919), Aloys Alzheimer (1864–1915), beide auch später auf neuropsychiatrischen Lehrstühlen sowie Walter Spielmeyer (1879–1935) und Willibald Scholz (1889–1917). Weiter wirkten auch Carl Weigert (1845–1904) in Frankfurt, Richard Paul Flechsig (1847–1929) in Leipzig, dort auch später Richard Arwed Pfeiffer (1858–1945) und schließlich Alfons Jakob (1884–1931) in Hamburg erfolgreich für die Neuropathologie.

Als letztes muß das Lebenswerk von Ludwig Edinger (1855–1918) besonders hervorgehoben werden, der wieder – wie viele vor ihm – als praktizierender Nervenarzt in Frankfurt begann. Auch er hat zunächst aus eigenen Mitteln ein neurologisches Institut aufgebaut, das heute noch in seiner alten Form im Rahmen der Universität als Stiftung erhalten ist.

Neben den aus der Neurologie und Psychiatrie stammenden Neuropathologen dürfen wir die aus der Allgemeinpathologie stammenden Wissenschaftler mit ihren wertvollen Beiträgen zur Neurologie nicht vergessen: Rudolf Virchow (1821–1902), den Erforscher der Glia und der Gliome, Julius Friedrich Cohnheim (1839–1884) mit seinen Studien zum Hirnkreislauf und schließlich Friedrich Daniel von Recklinghausen (1833–1919) mit seiner Geschwulstforschung und manch andere. Ihre Namen sind aus den Annalen der Neuropathologie nicht fortzudenken.

Welche Bedeutung diese Zusammenballung von weltbekannten Wissenschaftlern in der deutschen Neuropathologie gehabt hat, mag aus einem Zitat von Webb Haymaker hervorgehen, der schreibt: „Es ist keine Übertreibung zu sagen, daß in den letzten 50 Jahren

Deutschland in der morphologischen Neuropathologie die Welt geführt hat und vielleicht auch heute noch auf diesem Gebiet führend ist."

Das war im Jahre 1954.

Die Experimentellen Neurochirurgen und Neurochirurgen

Vergessen wir auch nicht die Beiträge der quasi-experimentell arbeitenden Neuropsychiater, wie Theodor Fritsch (1838–1927) und Eduard Hitzig (1838–1907) (Berlin), wie auch der ersten neurochirurgisch arbeitenden Chirurgen, wie Fedor Krause (1857–1937) (Berlin) für die Grundlagen der Neurologie.

Die neurologische Fachgesellschaften – Die Publikationsorgane

Kehren wir zurück zur deutschen Neurologie. Welche Organisationsform hatte sich nun dieses Fach für seine Mitglieder geschaffen? Von Erb, Oppenheim u. a. wurde 1907 die Gründung der „Gesellschaft Deutscher Nervenärzte" angeregt, die besonders in den späteren Jahren unter der Präsidentschaft von Max Nonne und Otfrid Foerster denkwürdige Kongresse abhalten konnte.

Nicht zu gering waren an den Erfolgen der Neurologie auch die literarischen Medien beteiligt gewesen, besonders der Beitrag des Springer-Verlages in Heidelberg mit der Betreuung fast aller neurologischen Zeitschriften. Diese waren: „Die Deutsche Zeitschrift für Nervenheilkunde" (gegründet 1891), jetzt als „Zeitschrift für Neurologie" bzw. „Journal of Neurology" fortgeführt, das "Archiv für Psychiatrie und Nervenkrankheiten" (1868), die „Zeitschrift für Neurologie und Psychiatrie" (1910), „Der Nervenarzt" (1928) und das „Zentralblatt für Neurologie und Psychiatrie" (1921). Diese Zeitschriften zeugen von der breiten Unterstützung, die unser Fach durch diesen Verlag erfahren hat, wozu noch die ausführliche Wiedergabe der neurologischen Kongreßberichte kam. Vergessen wir darüber nicht die „Springer-Handbücher": das erste Handbuch der Neurologie von Lewandowski (1910–1912) mit 5 Bänden und 2 Ergänzungsbänden und das von Bumke und Foerster herausgegebene Handbuch der Neurologie in 17 Bänden, welches 1936 vollendet wurde; es galt für lange Zeit als die „Bibel" für den Neurologen.

Diese Werke haben für die Welt den Stil eines „Handbuches" geprägt. Schließlich kam dazu die Reihe der „Monographien aus dem Gesamtgebiet der Neurologie und Psychiatrie" (1912): sie alle zeugen von der breiten und großherzigen Mitwirkung an unserem Fach durch den Heidelberger Verlag. In den letzten Jahrzehnten ist dazu noch eine weitere Zeitschrift „Aktuelle Neurologie" im Thieme-Verlag gekommen.

Die Deutsche Gesellschaft für Neurologie verleiht als höchste Auszeichnung die 1910 gestiftete Wilhelm Erb-Gedenkmünze (Abb. 10).

Hier soll noch eine kleine bezeichnende Anekdote folgen: Die besondere Struktur und die „Philosophie" der 3 deutschen großen Neurologen dieser Jahrzehnte: Max Nonne, Otfrid Foerster und Viktor von Weizsäcker, zeichnet die folgende – gut erfundene – Geschichte, die man sich in den 30iger Jahren zu erzählen pflegte.

Da treffen sich zwei Ordinarien für Medizin auf einem Kongreß und während des Gesprächs fragt der eine den anderen, ... „Zu wem er seinen Sohn zur neurologischen Ausbildung schicken solle"... ‚Das sei doch klar', meinte der andere: Zunächst, sozusagen für die ‚Lehrlingsjahre', zu Max Nonne nach Hamburg. Dort wird er eine gute Nosologie lernen. Für die ‚Gesellenjahre' würde ich ihn zu Otfrid Foerster nach Breslau gehen lassen. Dort wird er sogleich präzise neurologisch untersuchen lernen; weiter, wie das Gehirn und das übrige Nervensystem genau funktionierten und wo ein Krankheitsprozeß exakt zu lokalisieren ist.

Für die ‚Meisterklasse' aber, muß er wohl zu Viktor von Weizsäcker nach Heidelberg gehen. Dort wird er das ‚Walten des menschlichen Geistes und seiner Neurosen' in der Psychosomatik-Lehre erfahren und die ‚Psychogenie der Krankheiten' erfassen. Dort wird er dann auch merken, daß das meiste über die exakten Strukturen und Funktionen, was er bisher gelernt hatte, so nicht stimmt. Danach hat der Junge dann das Zeug, ein großer Neurologe zu werden ..."

Der Einbruch der nationalsozialistischen Herrschaft

Trotzdem wäre es wohl zu einer stetigen Weiterentwicklung der Neurologie gekommen, wäre nicht 1933 eine neue katastrophale Schwächung durch die Diktatur Hitlers in unserem Lande eingetreten. Eine größere Zahl neurologischer Wissenschaftler und Ärzte mußte Deutschland verlassen, an der Spitze Kurt Goldstein. Unsere Fachgesellschaft, die „Gesellschaft Deutscher Nervenärzte" wurde aufgelöst. Sie durfte nur unter der Präsidentschaft von Heinrich Pette (Hamburg) als eine „Abteilung für Neurologie" in einer Zwangsehe mit den Psychiatern weiterleben.

Das Kriegsende brachte dazu noch den Verlust eines Drittels von Deutschland und die Teilung des Restes in zwei Staaten. Schließlich verlor die Neurologie das Otfrid Foerster-Institut in Breslau und das Kaiser-Wilhelm-Institut in Berlin-Buch. Wir alle erinnern, wie 1945 Deutschland zudem materiell völlig zerschlagen war und auch personell erst wieder regeneriert werden mußte.

Wiederaufbau in der Bundesrepublik Deutschland

Die deutsche Neurologie zeigte nach dem zweiten Weltkrieg nur 4 ordentliche Lehrstühle an den verbliebenen westdeutschen Universitäten.

Derart bescheiden war die akademische Stellung im westdeutschen Teilstaat noch nach dem zweiten Weltkrieg. Die Gründe dafür habe ich erklärt. Die Neurologie wurde um diese Zeit vorwiegend auf den neuropsychiatrischen Lehrstühlen der Universitäten vertreten, innere Kliniken, die sich ebenfalls „Nervenklinik" nannten, waren in der Minderzahl. Andererseits waren die beiden Möglichkeiten einer rascheren Entwicklung in Berlin an der Neurologie vorübergegangen. Die Lehrstühle der Neurologie waren besetzt durch Heinrich Pette (1887–1964) in Hamburg, Georges Schaltenbrand (1897–1979) in Würzburg, Paul Vogel (1900–1979) in Heidelberg und durch Viktor von Weizsäcker (1886–1957), der nach dem

Verlust von Breslau nach Heidelberg auf einen Lehrstuhl für Allgemeine klinische Medizin 1945 zurückberufen wurde.

In der Folge wuchs zwar die Zahl der Neurologischen Lehrstühle (Tübingen, Freiburg, Düsseldorf usw.), die Masse der deutschen Ordinariate aber war noch immer mit Neuropsychiatern besetzt.

Dann aber mehrten sich immer mehr die Stimmen in der Neurologie, die eine Errichtung reiner neurologischer Lehrstühle für jede Universität forderten. Es wurde deshalb im Jahre 1962 auf dem Jahreskongreß in Köln, eine Diskussion über die Stellung der Neurologie vorbereitet. Wir wollten die Stellung unseres Faches in der Medizin umreißen und abgrenzen. Wir stellten die Trennung von der Psychiatrie zur Diskussion. Als Präsident dieses Kongresses hatte Paul Bucy aus Chicago als Neurochirurgen und Ludo van Bogaert und Frauchiger als Neurologen und Neuropathologen zu Referaten zu diesem Thema gebeten. Sie wurden durch fünf grundlagenwissenschaftliche Referate über die Sondergebiete der Neurologie ergänzt (Bauer, Behrend, Creutzfeld, Erbslöh, Glees).

Der Neuropsychiater Zutt hatte sich zu einer Stellungnahme zu diesem Thema bereit erklärt, hielt ein geschliffenes Referat, lehnte dann allerdings eine Diskussion aus Zeitmangel ab. Diese Diskussion ist dann von der jüngeren Generation fortgesetzt und im „Nervenarzt" veröffentlicht worden (s. Behrend et al. 1962) ebenso wie eine ausführliche Stellungnahme von Zutt über das Modell eines „Nervenzentrums". Dieses „Nervenzentrum" in Frankfurt ist aber nie zum Leben gebracht worden (Zutt, 1962, 1964).

Ohne weitere Diskussion hat dann seit 1963 die Wirklichkeit die Problematik überholt, in Westdeutschland ist die Trennung der Neurologie von der Psychiatrie auf den Lehrstühlen inzwischen weitgehend vollzogen.

Der Status der Neurologie in der Bundesrepublik

Wir haben jetzt in Westdeutschland etwa 220 neurologische Abteilungen, diese Zahl wächst stetig. Von diesen sind bis jetzt 172 auch statistisch durch Fragebogen von unserer Gesellschaft genauer analysiert. Es gibt an allen Universitäten insgesamt 33 selbständige Lehrstühle für Neurologie mit Klinik. Damit ist die „Neurologie" ein auch akademisch völlig selbständiges Fach geworden, wenn auch für den praktizierenden Nervenarzt neben dem „Gebietsarzt für Neurologie" oder „Psychiatrie" auch ein solcher für „Neuropsychiatrie" vorgesehen ist.

Nach dem Krieg ist die „Deutsche Gesellschaft für Neurologie" gegründet worden. Sie hat neben ihren Jahreskongressen in mehrjährigem Abstand einen gemeinsamen Kongreß mit ihren Nachbarfächern unter dem Schild der „Deutschen Gesellschaft für Psychiatrie und Nervenheilkunde".

Die Neurologie im Feld der neurologischen Wissenschaften

Blicken wir jetzt zusammenfassend auf die Stellung der Neurologie in der medizinischen Fakultät so ist zu sagen, daß wir in Freundschaft mit den Nachbarfächern leben. Mit der Inneren Medizin verbindet die moderne Neurologie sehr viel: von der Kreislauf-, Stoffwechsel- und Immun-Pathologie bis zur Organisation und Führung der Intensivstation. Entsprechend gut ist auch das Verhältnis zur Neurochirurgie, da kein Neurologe mehr auf die Idee kommen könnte, selbst das Messer in die Hand zu nehmen, abgesehen von einzelnen besonders begabten Kollegen, die die Stereotaxie durchführen. Die Grundlagenfächer Neuropathologie und das technische Fach der Neuroradiologie, haben sich weitgehend selbständig entwickelt. Daß gerade auf dem Felde der Neuroradiologie sich noch besonders viele Neurologen interessiert zeigen, geht darauf zurück, daß Neuroradiologie ja eigentlich nur eine Anatomie und Pathologie des Nervensystems mit besonderer Form der Abbildung ist. Wenn auch viele von uns in der Diagnostik noch gerne mitarbeiten, so wird auch hier keiner auf die Idee kommen, im technischen Bereich eine Aufgabe übernehmen zu wollen, geschweige denn in der therapeutischen Neuroradiologie mit dem Katheter (Interventionelle Neuroradiologie), die sich in den letzten Jahren so glänzend entwickelt hat. Wir glauben aber auch, daß das Verhältnis zur Psychiatrie gut ist.

Mir scheint, daß rein sachlich mit der Psychiatrie kaum Kompetenzschwierigkeiten entstehen können, wenn auch an einzelnen kleineren Abteilungen der Peripherie, die vollkommene Trennung von Neurologie und Psychiatrie organisatorisch noch nicht erfolgt ist.

Das große Gebiet der „Gehirnpathologie" im Sinne von Karl Kleist, d. h. die Neuropsychologie und ihre pathologischen Störungen, wird von beiden Fächern gleichmäßig und fruchtbar vertreten; das wird auch der diesjährige Weltkongreß erneut beweisen.

Nun wird heute mancher nach meiner Darstellung über die anfangs fast explosionsartige Entwicklung der Deutschen Wissenschaft und besonders der Neurologie fragen, wie es doch zu einem Absinken der Leistung im deutschen Raum gekommen ist. Die wirtschaftliche Situation kann es nicht sein, denn der Wiederaufbau nach dem 2. Weltkriege mit dem vielgepriesenen „Wirtschaftswunder", hatte sicher Mitte 1965 schon zu einem technischen Stand der Universitäten und Forschungsstätten geführt, der weit über dem nach dem 1. Weltkrieg in der sogenannten „Weimarer Republik" stand.

Damals mußte sogar eine „Notgemeinschaft der Deutschen Wissenschaft" gegründet werden, um überhaupt ein Überleben zu ermöglichen. Politische Unruhen, wirtschaftliche Katastrophen, Arbeitslosigkeit, waren viel drückender als nach diesem 2. Weltkriege. Erst eine genauere seelische Analyse der Generation nach 1968 – in der ganzen „technologischen" Welt – besonders aber in Deutschland nach der Nazi-Diktatur – wird uns den Schlüssel dazu geben. An den wirtschaftlich-technischen Möglichkeiten kann es nicht liegen.

Gibt es eine Krise der Neurologie?

Ich bin am Ende meiner historischen Übersicht. Wenn Sie diese etwa mit meinem Einleitungskapitel zum „Handbook of Clinical Neurology" (1969) vergleichen dann wird Ihnen auffallen, daß ich jetzt kaum von möglichen „Krisen" in der Neurologie gesprochen habe, die damals in der Diskussion noch einen großen Platz einnahmen.

Die meisten dieser Krisen haben sich seit den 60er Jahren von selber erledigt. Wenn ich zunächst zwei Punkte herausstelle, so betreffen sie die augenblickliche Struktur des Faches, ein dritter – mehr allgemeiner – Punkt erscheint jedoch ebenfalls drängend. Ich sehe die Hauptschwäche im Status der Deutschen Neurologie in den folgenden zwei Punkten:

1. Der Ausbildungsplan sieht – als Folge früherer Anschauungen über das Bild einer „Neuropsychiatrie" – eine fast 50%ige Ausbildung in der Psychiatrie vor, aber keinen Tag in der Inneren Medizin. Ich halte das bei der Struktur des Krankengutes einer neurologischen Klinik mit dem Einstrom der Kranken mit Hirn-, Kreislauf- und Stoffwechselstörungen für ein Unding.

2. Jede rasche strukturelle Vergrößerung eines Faches, bringt die große Gefahr der Verflachung der Ausbildung und verlangt eine fachliche Nachbesserung, z. B. durch Gründung einer jährlich tagenden (praktischen) Akademie für Neurologie, wie sie in den USA mit gutem Erfolg arbeitet. Diese ist dringend.

3. Ein dritter Punkt aber ist von allgemeinerer Bedeutung: Der Weltkrongreß 1985 wird zeigen, daß in unserem Interessenkreis die bildgebenden Verfahren – das Neuroimaging – eine große Rolle spielen. Die technischen Apparaturen gehören noch an vielen Orten in den Bereich der neurologischen oder neurochirurgischen Klinik, z. B. die Computertomographie (CT). Die Positron-Emissionstomographie (PET) und die neuromagnetischen Resonanzverfahren (NMR) sind noch so selten vertreten, daß die endgültige Position noch nicht ausgehandelt ist.

Aber die große Bedeutung dieser Verfahren, besonders des CT und des NMR, auch für die praktisch-klinische Diagnostik, haben uns erneut und immer dringlicher auf ein Problem hingewiesen: die Stellung der *apparativen* Diagnostik – wozu ich auch die inzwischen hochkomplizierten laborchemischen Untersuchungen rechne – im Bereich der neurologischen Untersuchung. Deren Position halte ich für einen wichtigen Diskussionspunkt.

Es ist ein billiges Alltagsthema unserer Medien und des Laienpublikums festzustellen, daß das Patienten-Arzt-Vertrauen immer mehr schwindet, daß die Patienten von den Ärzten vielfach enttäuscht seien. Woher kommt denn das? Einige der wichtigen Ursachen sind z.B. die Abkürzung der Zeit, die wir mit den Patienten verbringen, weil die körperliche Untersuchung immer mehr hinter den technischen Untersuchungsmethoden zurücktritt, während diese tatsächlich zu Überwuchern beginnen. Aus der Arzt-Patienten-Beziehung, wird die Person des behandelnden Arztes immer mehr durch die Technologie verdrängt. Gewiß haben die Fortschritte der apparativen und Laboratiums-Diagnostik die Therapie in erstaunlichem Maße verbessert. Daß sie aber oft *ohne* strenge Indikation, *zu früh* und deshalb wohl auch *zu häufig* eingesetzt werden, haben wir zu wenig erkannt.

Bedenken wir doch: In vielen Fällen einer neurologischen Erkrankung kann auch heute noch eine gute Digagnose durch die genügend genaue Anamnese und die körperlich-neurologische Untersuchung gestellt werden, oder zumindesten erlaubt sich eine gefestigte Verdachtsdiagnose. Dieser Teil der Untersuchung ist verhältnismäßig rasch durchgeführt, er ist einfach und billig. Zudem aber schafft er – und das ist wichtig – die Bekanntschaft zwischen Arzt und Patienten und damit das nötige Vertrauensverhältnis.

Gewiß kann man die großen Erfolge der apparativen Untersuchung gar nicht genügend würdigen, sie *müssen* angewandt werden. Doch ist es oft der Patient selbst, der den *allzu frühzeitigen* Einsatz des „Apparates" fordert.

Die Verschiebung der Diagnostik zum Technologischen hin, ist nicht neu, sie ist nicht auf die Neurologie beschränkt. Viktor von Weizsäcker, der selbst aus der Inneren Medizin kam, pflegte immer etwas verächtlich von dem Überwuchern des „Zettelkataloges" am Krankenbett des Patienten in der Inneren Medizin zu sprechen, in dem die Ergebnisse des Labors und der Apparate festgehalten wurden.

In diesem Spannungsfeld leben also heute in der Medizin die meisten Ärzte, zumindest in den hochtechnisierten Ländern.

Unsere Pflicht aber ist es zu versuchen das Vertrauensverhältnis zwischen Arzt und Patienten wiederzugewinnen. In der Neurologie wäre das relativ einfach zu erreichen, kehrten wir zur genauen körperlichen Untersuchung zurück. Eine gute neurologische Befragung und Untersuchung dauert einige Zeit. Viktor von Weizsäcker pflegte zu sagen: „Ein gutes halbes Stündchen".

Sicher wird in diesem Augenblick der Diskussion der Einwand kommen: wer denn wohl in dem hektischen Betrieb des Kassenarztes diese Zeit noch aufbringen könne? Aber wir müssen einen Weg finden, um das Vertrauensverhältnis zum Patienten wiederzufinden, das heutzutage brüchig zu werden beginnt.

Auch die folgenden Gesichtspunkte sind von Bedeutung: Große Teile Europas und der dritten Welt verfügen gar nicht – aus wirtschaftlichen Gründen – über eine ausgedehnte apparative Diagnostik, die uns so große Erfolge gebracht hat. Wir aber müssen lernen, diese Apparate in der richtigen Reihenfolge und mit der richtigen Fragestellung anzuwenden. Computertomographie und Kernspin stehen nicht am Anfang der neurologischen Untersuchung, sondern eher am Ende – außer natürlich in der Notfalldiagnostik!

Wir sprachen von dem Überwuchern der apparativen Diagnostik, sie ist doch zu einem nicht unerheblichen Teil an der Kostenexplosion in unserer Medizin beteiligt, von der wir ja erdrückt werden. Stellen wir das fest, so wird man uns hoffentlich nicht vorwerfen, wir predigten jetzt die Rückkehr zur „guten alten Zeit"; man wird vielleicht auch betonen, dieser Teil der Diagnostik sei doch rascher und sicherer. Die Apparate *sollen* auch eingesetzt werden, aber nur bei guter Indikation, gewonnen nach ärztlicher Untersuchung mit genauer Anamnese.

Hier ist aber zu betonen, daß auch die Computertomographie und manche andere apparative Methode durch falsche Ausdeutung zu Fehldiganosen führen kann und zwar aufgrund mangelnder Daten einer klinischen Voruntersuchung. Diese hätte bei genauer Indikationsstellung, guter Anamnese und neurologischem Befund, vermieden werden können.

Daher sollten wir als Neurologen aus dieser Diskussion einen Leitsatz mitnehmen dürfen: Wir dürfen das „alte Rüstzeug" der genauen neurologischen Untersuchung nicht vergessen, das uns auch wieder auf den richtigen Weg des engeren Vertrauensverhältnisses zum Patienten bringen wird.

Wohin uns Ärzte am Ende dieses Jahrhunderts der Weg noch

führen wird, wir wissen es nicht. Bei der früheren Bearbeitung dieses Themas (1969) wurden dazu einige Gedanken geäußert, die allerdings weitgehend Phantasie geblieben sind. Percival Bailey hat einmal gesagt: Wir Neurologen sollten auch einmal träumen können. Träumen wir also von einer hoffentlich heileren Welt und einem angemessenen und kontrollierten Fortschritt, den wir dann aus ganzem Herzen bejahen. An diesem wollen wir dann auch mit ganzer Kraft arbeiten.

Ich bin am Ende meines Berichtes und wünsche Ihnen einen guten Kongreßverlauf in der Stadt Hamburg und in dem Lande, dessen Geschichte der Neurologie ich versuchte Ihnen darzustellen.

Historical Development of German Neurology

Speech for the Opening of the World Congress of Neurology in Hamburg, 1985

Mr. Mayor, Chairmen and Secretaries, Ladies and Gentlemen.

We are delighted that you, neurologists from all over the world, have come to Germany for your World Congress in 1985; this is the first time in the history of neurology and it is a particular honour for Hamburg, the place of influence of Max Nonne, one of our famous neurologists; indeed, it was he who headed the first neurological Department (1896) here in the old Eppendorf Hospital, built in 1884, and held the first chair of pure Neurology when the University of Hamburg was founded in 1919.

To open the conference, I should like to tell you about the development of German neurology. To start with, I shall describe the general picture of the neurological sciences at the turn of the 18th century by referring to several prominent neurologists of that time. It was then that medicine slowly began to turn to the natural sciences for its basis.

Let us recall: a century previously, the term "neurology" had been first coined by Thomas Willis (1622–1675): he introduced "neurologia" as an independent discipline, in addition to "osteologia" and "myologia". Which particular lines did then this new science of neurology emphasize a century later?

By the turn of the 18th century, Marshall Hall (1790–1875) had developed his theory of reflexes, James Parkinson (1755–1824) had

---

My particular thanks go to Dr. Helen Cooper for the excellent translation of the German text.

described shaking palsy as a uniform clinical picture and Charles Bell (1747–1842) had comprehended the function of the spinal roots. Further, Francois Magendie (1783–1842) had succeeded in elucidating the actions of the spinal cord and Jean Cruveilhier (1791–1874) had published his excellent "Atlas of Pathological Anatomy of the Nervous System". In Italy, Giovanni Battista Morgagni (1682–1771) had described the first pathological foundation of diseases for all areas (e. g. apoplexy) and Luigi Galvani (1737–1798) had shown that electric currents can arise from muscle activity. The gifted polymath, Alexander von Humboldt (1769–1859) was able to exploit these findings in his experimental studies. This led to the founding of nerve physiology. But otherwise, at this time in Germany, only Johann Christian Reil (1759–1843) was well-known; he had outlined an overall first concept regarding the cooperation between individual parts of the brain. Finally, Samuel Thomas Soemmering (1755–1830) had shown the brain to be the organ of the mind and had correctly classified the cranial nerves.

Fundamental Changes in Berlin: the Founding of the University

These were some of the most important scientific achievements which, like the stones of a mosaic, led to a picture of nervous system functions. But now, during the first third of the 19th century, there suddenly appeared in Berlin a generation of young research workers on the scientific stage, stimulated by an anatomist who later became a physiologist, namely, Johannes Müller (1801–1858) (Fig. 1), a student of Asmund Rudolphi (1771–1831). Müller had been called to take up the Chair in Berlin at the age of only 31. He ended the founding of medicine on "natural philosophy". Only a few years later, he published a "Handbook of Physiology" in which he developed a fascinating picture of the nervous functions of man and animals. From those who were direct students of his, only a few can be mentioned here: Theodor Schwann (1810–1885) who soon left for Belgium to take up the Chair at Loewen, Friedrich Gustav Jakob Henle (1809–1885) who was appointed to the Chair in Zürich,

Heinrich Friedrich Bidder (1810–1884) who returned to the German University of Dorpat, and finally Heinrich Remak (1815–1865) who remained in Berlin and indeed taught a whole generation of anatomists. But the number of students and colleagues of Johannes Müller was much larger. Let us mention the physiologists Du Bois-Reymond (1818–1896), Carl Ludwig (1816–1895) and Ernst Brücke (1819–1892), and the anatomists Albert Koelliker (1817–1905), Friedrich Leopold Goltz (1834–1902) and the gifted Hermann von Helmholtz (1821–1894), over whom it was long argued whether he belonged to the ophthalmologists, the physiologists or the anatomists. Even Rudolf Virchow, the pathologist (1821–1902), and the surgeon Theodor Billroth (1829–1894), Privat-Dozent in Berlin and later called to take up the Chair in Vienna, as well as the scientist Ernst Haeckel (1824–1912), well known for his involvement in discussions with Darwin, have all called themselves students of Johannes Müller. Also Otto Loewy, already called to join the faculty in Graz as Privat-Dozent, belonged to those scientists who took their first step under Johannes Müller.

This remarkable growth of the Berlin Medical School, which produced such renowned and excellent scientists in a relatively short time after the effective "vacuum" of the 18th century, is quite amazing. Probably it can be understood only in the context of this period, the main features of which I now quickly want to sketch.

Europe had just been freed from Napoleon's rule. The uprising in Prussia was initiated by speeches from Fichte and Schleiermacher in Berlin who knew how to inspire the young people intellectually to fight for the freedom of Europe. Wilhelm von Humboldt (1809) joined them as director of education; he had laid proposals before the king for a new model of a university in which the professors should be free of state influence and able to devote themselves equally to both research *and* teaching.

As a preliminary step towards such a university, he founded the "gymnasium" as the more elevated educational school. The king followed the recommendation for the founding of the university in Berlin and stressed, in 1811: "Now we must replace, with intellectual powers, that which has been lost physically." In Prussia the climate was ripe for the fight against the Napoleonic regime and for a free democracy. Nonetheless, the youth in Europe was subsequently betrayed in its democratic ideals of freedom by the "reaction" which prevailed in the mid-European countries following the Vienna Congress. In vain had some of the new academics taken to the streets to protest together with the students. However, at the universities, the enthusiasm was largely transmuted from its political nature to produce astounding successes in science.

But also as a consequence remained the suppression of the wished-for liberty, which led to the well-known political revolt of the years 1832 and 1848.

Moritz-Heinrich Romberg, the First Neurological Clinician

But for neurology there came a new phenomenon in the form of the young internist Moritz-Heinrich Romberg (1786–1873) (Fig. 2). In 1840 he became the Director of the Royal Policlinical Institute in Berlin. It is amazing that already that same year he was able to begin with the publication of his clinical experience in the first volume of his "Textbook of Nervous Diseases in Man". This book was immediately translated into English and shortly thereafter began to exert its influence in England and America. Just how much Kalinowski and Houston Merrit/USA (1954) rate the importance of this young neurologist is shown by the fact that they view the setting-up of Romberg's clinic as the "beginning of neurology". Ramsey Hunt (USA) too describes Romberg's textbook as the "first systematic description of neurology" in internal medicine (1933/34).

Apparently this first rousing publication in the new field exerted a fruitful influence on the remaining Germany where we can now see the great clinicians of this century developing – Nikolaus Friedreich (1825–1882) in Würzburg and Heidelberg (Fig. 3), Adolf Kussmaul (1822–1902) in Erlangen, Ernst Leyden (1832–1919) in Berlin, Adolf Strümpell (1856–1925) in Leipzig (Fig. 4), Friedrich Schultze (1845–1935) in Göttingen, Paul Julius Möbius (1853–1907) in Leipzig, Ludwig Traube (1818–1876) in Berlin and Heinrich Curschmann d. Ä. (1846–1910) in Hamburg and Leipzig.

Contributions of Fundamental Research to Neurology

But the flame spread to the other basic neurological sciences and created a new enthusiasm for scientific work which now tended to be founded on *general pathology*. I mention here Friedrich Daniel von Recklinghausen (1833–1910), Julius Friedrich Cohnheim (1839–1884), Carl Weigert (1845–1904) and the great Rudolf Virchow (1821–1902) who set a worldwide example for this century by providing a new and now pathogenetically oriented clinic, controlled by the pathologists.

Representatives of *normal anatomy and physiology* joined forces with this forward-looking movement: Albert Koelliker (1863–1905), Wilhelm His (1831–1904), Michael von Lenhossék in Würzburg (1863–1937) and Johann Purkinje (1787–1869) in Breslau are worthy representatives of their fields. The latter was called from the Karls'University in Prague, where he held the post of Prosector, to Breslau. Here he developed the first modern institute of physiology in the world.

We can well see that now young gifted scientists from neighbouring countries pressed to enter the German universities because of their excellent working conditions and their correspondingly stimulating atmosphere.

The Further Development in Berlin

Thus passed the 19th century in Berlin and the remainder of Germany. But what now follwed the exceptionally fortuitous start to neurology, under Moritz Romberg, during the change to the 20th century? Was it still possible to catch up with the successes gained by our British neighbours – represented by Victor Horsley, C. E. Beevor, Marcus Gunn, Charlton Bastian, Hughlings Jackson, W. R. Gowers and David Ferrier, and finally Charles E. Brown-Sèquard – at the National Hospital, Queen's Square, and by the French at the Salpetrière with Charcot, Broca, Dejerine, Babinski and later Pierre Marie, namely, to found a leading institute for neurology in the capital? No – that proved not possible: it was disappointing to see just what happened in Berlin.

The outstanding Wilhelm Griesinger (1817–1868) was in fact appointed as successor to Romberg; but he, as a psychiatrist, had developed a mammoth programme for the modernisation and humanisation of psychiatry. In Berlin, he received, in addition to the Romberg's Poliklinisches-Institut which was largely oriented in a neurological direction, his own psychiatric department at the Charité. But most of the neurology landed, with internal medicine, in the hands of Ernst von Leyden (1832–1910). Sadly, Griesinger was not able to realize his humanitarian programme in Berlin: he died young, and a student of Romberg, Karl Westphal (1833–1890) became his successor.

But Westphal too developed an incurable illness and from then on, until his death, Hermann Oppenheim, his favourite student, acted as his provisional representative. He was finally put forward by the Faculty unico loco as successor but the Ministry did not concur, because of his creed, an event which understandably caused him to be bitter. He was, after all, one of the first "pure" neurologists and was now faced with only one course open to him, namely, to resign from the university. He nevertheless maintained an out-patient clinic and a laboratory from his own finances and remained so well-known that neurological patients streamed to him from all over the world.

In 1896, Hermann Oppenheim was able to publish his "Textbook of Neurology", the compilation of which had proved exhausting. But it had the effect of making him known throughout the world: Seven German, three English and one each of Russian, Spanish and Italian editions followed – Oppenheim really became "Praeceptor mundi" in neurology. Nevertheless, Oppenheim could not get over the fact that he had been forced to leave the University. And thereby a decisive moment in the development of neurology in Germany had been missed, simply because Oppenheim, the most famous German neurologist, had not been called to the confluence point in Berlin.

Once again, later, a second opportunity arose to develop neurology further in Berlin and Germany: The psychiatrist Emil Kraepelin (1856–1926) was called from Munich to take the vacant professorial chair in Berlin in 1912. Kraepelin was widely known from his textbook of the first nosological classification of psychiatry. He accepted the appointment, but on one condition, namely, that simultaneously neurology be separated from psychiatry and that it be given a department with its own chair and an associated clinic. But this proposal was rejected by the Berliner Ministry.

Instead, Karl Bonhoeffer (1868–1948) was called from Breslau. He, like his teacher Wernicke, must be viewed as one of the advocates of "neuropsychiatry". For Bonhoeffer too, diseases of the mind were "diseases of the brain", just as for Griesinger and Karl Wernicke (1848–1905). They were the first clear marked leaders of such a field of neuropsychiatry, as represented later in Germany by Hoche, Bumke, Karl Kleist, Binswanger and Berger. Neurology remained at the universities – with few exceptions – in the hands of these neuropsychiatrists.

Had a Chair of Neurology been created in Berlin at that time, the direction of the development of German neurology would have been set. But that did not take place. Now the second and last "chance" for German neurology had been lost. We shall later describe the subsequent catastrophic development after 1933.

Neurology in Internal Medicine

In the meantime, we must catch up on what had happened to neurology in the confines of internal medicine. What arose from this root? The internist Wilhelm Erb (1840–1921) in Heidelberg (Fig. 5), exceedingly interested in neurology and with an excellent knowledge of muscle diseases and of electrotherapy and electropathology, was the decisive figure here. As Professor of Internal Medicine, he had made a clear decision for himself: "the field of 'Nervenpathologie' – as he at that time named neurology – was too broad, he wrote, to be represented together with internal medicine by *one* scientist."

Erb expounded in one of his major speeches (1880), "that it is not necessary any longer to present extensive evidence that the real scientific and fruitful investigation of nerve pathology can be provided by anyone other than a specialitst, utter devotion, and all the working energy of one man is necessary in order to have at least some command of this enormous field. How much more is needed to deal with it independently and productively..." This view was one that Erb continually put forward at conferences over decades.

As a consequence, it proved indeed to be the case that German neurology – in contrast to many other countries – later had less difficulty in separating itself from internal medicine.

Neurology in General Hospitals

But what then happened to neurology? Strangely enough, much support for this field came from the efforts of important figures working in the large municipal hospitals. This contribution was really not unimportant for the development of German neurology. Thus in Hannover (Ludwig Bruns, 1858–1916), in Dortmund (only temporarily), in Danzig (Adolf Wallenberg, 1862–1939) and in Breslau (Ludwig Mann, 1866–1936, in addition to Otfrid Foerster, 1873–1941) (Fig. 7) municipal departments were successfully set up. Above I have already mentioned the activities of Max Nonne (1861–1959) in Hamburg (Fig. 6), who as early as 1896 created his own neurological clinic in the General Hospital Eppendorf. Max Nonne succeeded in establishing neurological departments under former students of his in all large hospitals in Hamburg. It is probably for this reason that clinical neurology in West Germany is most densely represented in Hamburg.

Furthermore, I want to point here especially to the neurological activities of Otfrid Foerster who managed to set up, within the neurological clinic in a municipal hospital, a special department for patients suffering from brain injuries and later even to build up a "Neurological Research Institute" which became known worldwide.

The Famous Neurological Research Institutes

Otfrid Foerster (1873–1941) in Breslau (Fig. 7) was indeed the most important neurologist Germany ever produced. He was also equally regarded by the neurosurgeons. Most American older emeritus neurosurgeons of the present have spent some time at the Neurological Research Institute in Breslau with Otfrid Foerster, some of the most prominent being Percival Bailey, Paul Bucy, Wilder Penfield and Josef P. Evans. For a long time, Otfrid Foerster could only maintain his laboratory at a municipal hospital from his personal means. Only in 1932 did the Rockefeller Foundation – following the recommendation of American friends – build the modern neurological research institute together with the state of Prussia and the city of Breslau. But by that time it was really already too late – the major part of the life's work of Otfrid Foerster had been completed. Under his successor in Breslau, Viktor von Weizsäcker (Fig. 8) (1886–1957), the institute gained the name "Otfrid Foerster-Institute".

The second most notable personality in the circle of neurological clinicians and fundamental research workers was Oskar Vogt (1876–1959), who, together with his wife Cécile, created the large Kaiser-Wilhelm-Institut in Berlin-Buch (Fig. 9). He too had to wait for two decades for this new building, but similarly he had to start with a small laboratory – set up from his own means.

From the famous Berlin Institute came: Korbinian Brodmann (1868–1918) and Max Bielschowsky (1869–1940) as well as Timofjejew, the geneticist; later Hugo Spatz (1888–1969) took over the directorship and succeeded in gaining Julius Hallervorden (1882–1965) and Wilhelm Tönnis (1898–1978) as outstanding colleagues. But here too, as in Breslau with Otfrid Foerster and in Munich with Emil Kraepelin – at the Research Institute for Psychiatry – it was first the Rockefeller Foundation which, by dint of generous support, made possible the setting up of a large research institute in Berlin-Buch.

These three institutes came to form a considerable support for the development of the neurological sciences and became a Mecca, especially in the field of neuropathology, for the training of many young scientists from all over the world. As a result of the last war, however, Breslau and Berlin-Buch became lost for neurology.

The Neuropathologists

We have just mentioned the neuropathologists working in Berlin-Buch and must now particularly underline the people working at the Munich Kaiser-Wilhelm Institute for Psychiatry under Emil Kraepelin (1856–1926): Franz Nissl (1860–1919), Aloys Alzheimer (1864–1915), – both later to occupy chairs in neuropsychiatry – as well as Walter Spielmeyer (1879–1935) and Willibald Scholz (1889–1917).

Other important figures as regards neuropathology were Carl Weigert (1845–1904) in Frankfurt, Richard Paul Flechsig (1847–1929) in Leipzig where also Richard Arwed Pfeiffer (1858–1945) was later, and finally Alfons Jakob (1884–1931) in Hamburg.

Lastly, the life's work of Ludwig Edinger (1855–1918) must be particularly stressed: he, as many before him, began as a practising "Nervenarzt" in Frankfurt. He too first financed his own neurological institute, which has been preserved until the present in its original form within the University as a Foundation.

In addition to those neuropathologists originating from neurology and psychiatry, we should not forget those scientists coming from general pathology and who made such valuable contributions to neurology: Rudolf Virchow (1821–1902), the person who researched into glia and gliomas, Julius Friedrich Cohnheim (1839–1884) with his studies on the circulation in the brain and finally Friedrich Daniel von Recklinghausen (1833–1919) who researched into tumours, as well as many others. Their names will continue to go down in the annals of neuropathology.

Of what importance this concentration of world-famous scientists in German neuropathology had, can be deduced from a quotation from Webb Haymaker: "it is no exaggeration to say that in the last fifty years Germany has led the world in morphological neuropathology and possibly is still today a leader in this field."

That was in 1954.

The Experimental Neurosurgeons and Neuropsychiatrists

Let us also not forget the contributions to fundamental neurology of the quasi-experimental neuropsychiatrists such as Theodor Fritsch (1838–1927) and Eduard Hitzig (1838–1907) (Berlin), nor the first neurosurgically-oriented surgeons such as Fedor Krause (1857–1937) (Berlin).

The Neurological Society – the Organs of Publication

We will here return to German neurology. Which form of organization had this field created for its members? Erb, Oppenheim and others suggested in 1907 that the "Gesellschaft Deutscher Nervenärzte" be founded, and which particularly in later years, under the presidency of Max Nonne and Otfrid Foerster, held memorable meetings.

The literary media were also not inconsiderably involved in the success of neurology, in particular the Springer Publishing House in Heidelberg contributed by looking after nearly all the neurological journals. The latter were: Die Deutsche Zeitschrift für Nervenheilkunde (founded in 1891), now known as the Zeitschrift für Neurologie or the Journal of Neurology, the Archiv für Psychiatrie und Nervenkrankheiten (1868), the Zeitschrift für Neurologie und Psychiatrie (1921). These journal demonstrate the broad support which our field has sustained from these publishers and which was added to by the detailed proceedings of neurological meetings. And do not let us forget thereby the "Springer Handbooks": the first Handbook of Neurology was by Lewandowski (1910–1912) and of five volumes and 2 supplementary volumes, and the Handbook of Neurology edited by Bumke and Foerster ran to 17 volumes and was completed in 1936 and regarded as the "Bible" for neurologists for a very long time. These works set the style of such handbooks; finally, in addition to those mentioned above, there came the series "Monographien aus dem Gesamtgebiet der Neurologie und Psychiatrie" (1912): they all illustrate the broad and generous support our field has had from the Heidelberg Verlag. During the last decade another journal "Aktuelle Neurologie" has appeared, published by Thieme.

The "Deutsche Gesellschaft für Neurologie" awards the "Erb Commemorative Medal" (Fig. 10), sponsored in 1910, as the highest prize.

The particular structure and the "philosophy" of the three great German neurologists of these decades. Max Nonne, Otfrid Foerster and Viktor von Weizsäcker, is illustrated by the following – well thought up – anecdote which was readily told during the 1930s:

Two Professors of Medicine meet at a congress and during the course of conversation, one asks the other... "to whom he should send his son for his neurological training... 'No doubt about it,' the other thought: firstly, for the time of his 'apprenticeship', to Max Nonne in Hamburg. There he would learn nosology well.

For his 'training' period, he should go to Otfrid Foerster in Breslau where he would learn precise neurological examination and further, exactly how the brain and the remaining nervous system functions and where a disease process can be exactly located. For the 'master class' though, he must go to Viktor von Weizsäcker in Heidelberg.

There he would gain experience in the 'workings of the human mind' and their neuroses in the science of psychosomatics and learn to understand the psychogeny of disease. There he would then also notice that most of the exact structures and functions of which he had learnt up till then were not true. Forthwith, the young man would be thus in a position to become a great neurologist..."

The Incursion of Nazi Rule

A steady growth in neurology could possibly still have taken place had there not been the catastrophic developments of 1933 with the dictatorship of Hitler. A large number of doctors and scientists had to leave Germany, at their head Kurt Goldstein. Our society, the "Gesellschaft Deutscher Nervenärzte" was dissolved and was permitted only to exist under the chairmanship of Heinrich Pette

(Hamburg) as a "Department of Neurology" in a new society and here in a forced marriage with the psychiatrists.

The end of the war brought with it the loss of one third of Germany and the division of the remainder into two countries. Finally, neurology lost the Otfrid-Foerster-Institut in Breslau and the Kaiser-Wilhelm-Institut in Berlin-Buch. We all remember just how, in 1945, Germany was in addition completely smashed materially and also how personnel also first had to be regenerated.

Recovery in the Bundesrepublik Following the War

German neurology had only four chairs at the West German universities remaining at the end of the Second World War. The academic position was still as modest after the War. I have explained the reasons for that. Neurology at this time was represented primarily by neuropsychiatric chairs at the universities, departments of clinics of internal medicine – which also called themselves "Nervenabteilungen" – were in a minority. Chairs in Neurology were occupied by Heinrich Pette (1887–1964) in Hamburg, Georges Schaltenbrand (1897–1979) in Würzburg, Paul Vogel (1900–1979) in Heidelberg and Viktor von Weizsäcker (1886–1957) who, after the loss of Breslau, was called back to Heidelberg to take up a Chair in General Clinical Medicine in 1945.

As a consequence, the number of neurological chairs did indeed increase (Tübingen, Freiburg, Düsseldorf etc.), but most of the German professorial chairs were still occupied by neuropsychiatrists.

But then the number of voices in neurology which were in favour of establishing purely neurological chairs in each university increased. For this reason, at the annual meeting in 1962 in Cologne, a discussion was prepared regarding the position of neurology. We wanted the position of our field within medicine to be clearly demarcated and separate and we raised the subject of partitioning neurology from psychiatry. As President of this congress, I had invited Paul Bucy from Chicago as a neurosurgeon and Ludo van Bogaert and Frauchiger as neurologists and neuropathologists to speak on this topic. Their talks were supplemented by fundamental scientific reports on special fields of neurology (Bauer, Behrend, Creutzfeld, Erbslöh, Glees).

The psychiatrist Zutt had said he was prepared to take up a position on this matter and held a highly polished talk; but then he declined any discussion owing to a lack of time. This discussion was then taken up by the younger generation and published in "Nervenarzt" (see Behrend et al. 1962) just as was an extensive commentary by Zutt on the model for a "Nervenzentrum". But this "Nervenzentrum" in Frankfurt never came to life (Zutt, 1962, 1964).

Without further discussion, reality has overtaken the problems since 1963; in the Bundesrepublik the separation of neurology from psychiatry in terms of professorial chairs has, in the meantime, been virtually completed.

The Status of Neurology in the Bundesrepublik

We now have about 220 departments of neurology in West Germany and this number is steadily growing. From these 220, some 172 have been analysed statistically, using questionaires, in more detail by our society. We have a total of 33 independent professorships in neurology which are attached to a clinic, thereby making "neurology" effectively a completely independent field academically-speaking, even if for the practising nerve specialist in addition to the "Gebietsarzt für Neurologie" or "Psychiatrie", there is also one for "Neuropsychiatrie".

After the War, the "Deutsche Gesellschaft für Neurologie" was successfully set up as successor to the former "Gesellschaft deutscher Nervenärzte". In addition to its annual meetings it holds, at intervals of a few years, a common conference with the neighbouring fields under the title "Deutsche Gesellschaft für Psychiatrie und Nervenheilkunde".

Neurology within the Neurological Sciences

If we now look summarily at the position of neurology in the medical faculty we can say that we live together as good neighbours with our bordering fields. Modern neurology is much connected to internal medicine: from circulatory, metabolic and immuno-pathology to the organisation and management of the intensive care unit. The relationship to neurosurgery is correspondingly good: no neurologist could any longer get the idea of taking the scalpel in his own hand, save for a few particularly gifted colleagues who perform stereotaxy. The fundamental field of neuropathology and neurophysiology and the technical field of neuroradiology have largely developed independently. That particularly many neurologists show interest in neuroradiology can be traced back to the fact that neuroradiology is really only an anatomy and pathology of the nervous system having an especial form of depiction. Even though many of us still willingly work in the field of diagnostics, here too no one would consider taking over a task falling in a technical area, let alone in therapeutic neuroradiology with a catheter (interventional neuroradiology) which has developed so glowingly over the past few years.

We also believe that our relations with psychiatry are good though it appears to me that we cannot run into difficulties on purely material grounds as regards competence, even though in individual small departments the complete separation of neurology and psychiatry has not yet been organizationally accomplished.

The large field of "brain pathology" in the sense adopted by Karl Kleist i. e. neuropsychology and its pathological disorders is represented by both fields equally and fruitfully; this year's World Congress will again prove that.

But now some may ask, after my account of the initially almost explosion-like development of German science and particularly neurology, just why it has come to some decline in performance in Germany. It can hardly be the economic situation, since following the Second World War the recovery, with its much admired "Wirtschaftswunder", had certainly already led, by the middle of 1965, to a technical status in the universities and research institutions that far exceeded that after the First World War in the so-called "Weimarer Republik". At that time a "Notgemeinschaft der Deutschen Wissenschaft" even had to be formed in order to survive at all. Political unrest, economic catastrophes, and unemployment were all much more oppressive than after this Second World War. Only a more exact analysis of the generation after 1968 – in the entire "technological" world – but especially in Germany following the Nazi dictatorship – will provide us with the key. It cannot be accounted for by the economic-technical opportunities.

Is there a Crisis in Neurology?

I am now at the end of my historical survey. If you compare it with my introductory chapter of the "Handbook of Clinical Neurology", then you will notice that here I have not mentioned possible general "crises" in neurology at all, whereas they were given considerable exposure in that discussion. But most of the crises dealt with there have resolved themselves since the sixties. If I first stress two points, these refer to the present structure of the field: a third – more general – point however appears to be similarly urgent. I see the main weaknesses as regards German neurology in the following two points:

1. Training involves – ass a consequence of earlier views about the picture of "neuropsychiatry" – about 50% of the time to be spent in psychiatric departments, but not one single day in internal medicine. I consider this absurd in view of the fact that the patient structure of a neurological clinic is such that it contains an influx of patients with brain, circulatory and metabolic etc. disorders.

2. Every rapid structural enlargement of a field brings with it the danger of a decline in training. That requires relevant subsequent improvement, for example by the founding of an Academy of Neurology which meets annually and as operates in the USA with a high degree of success.

3. A third point however is of general importance: the World Congress 1985 will show that in our sphere of interest, those methods

producing images – neuroimaging – play a major role. The technical devices still belong in many places to the area of the neurological or neurosurgical clinic, for example, computer tomography (CT). Positron emission tomography (PET) and neuromagnetic resonance methods (NMR) are still represented so rarely that they have not yet attained their final position.

But the enormous significance of these methods, in particular of CT and NMR, – for practical-clinical diagnosis too – have indicated afresh and increasingly urgently one problem: the position of apparatus-based diagnosis – to which I would also add the highly complicated chemical investigations performed in the laboratory – within the context of neurological examination. I consider this an important topic for discussion.

It is a common everyday topic arising in the media and discussed by the lay public that the relationship between doctor and patient is steadily diminishing and that patients are often disappointed by their doctors. Where does this attitude come from? Some of the most important aspects are, for example, the shortening of time available to be spent with patients, owing to the fact that the physical examination increasingly disappears into the background compared to the technical methods of examination; the latter, on the other hand, are starting to overgrow. The person behind the doctor treating the patient is increasingly being pushed out by technology from the doctor/patient relationship. There is no doubt that advances in apparatus-based and laboratory diagnosis have led to astounding improvements in the treatment of patients. But we have failed to acknowledge that they are often employed without any pressing indication, too early and thus also too often.

Let us consider: in many cases of neurological disease, a good diagnosis can still be made today on the basis of an adequately accurate anamnesis and a physical neurological examination, or at the least a firm suspected diagnosis can be made. This part of the examination can be performed relatively rapidly – added to which: it is simple and cheap. And furthermore, it creates – and that is important – a relationship between doctor and patient and thereby the necessary confidence.

Certainly one cannot pay enough tribute to the enormous successes of the apparatus-based examination – such examinations *must* be applied. But it is often the patient himself who demands the all too *premature* introduction of "technology".

The shift of diagnostics towards technology is not new and is not restricted to neurology. Viktor von Weizsäcker, who came from internal medicine, always used to speak there somewhat derogatively of the overgrowth found at the patient's bedside in "catalogues of notes" in which the results obtained from the laboratory and using apparatus were reported.

It is in this field of tension that most doctors, at least in highly technological countries, live today.

It is our duty however to try to regain the relationship between a doctor and his patients. In neurology that would be relatively simple to attain were we to return to the exact physical examination. But a well-conducted questioning and examination takes some time – Viktor von Weizsäcker used to say: "a good half hour". Certainly at present the objection will be raised: who on earth in the hectic practice of a general practitioner can still find that time today? But we *must* find a way to recover this relationship to patients which has already begun to crack.

The following points are also of significance: large areas of Europe and the developing countries do not have access – for economic reasons – to those extensive apparatus based diagnostics which have brought us so much success. But we must learn to apply these pieces of equipment in the right order and with the correct questions being born in mind. Computer tomography and nuclear spin resonance do not form the *beginning* of the neurological examination, but rather the *end* – except, of course, in emergency diagnosis!

We spoke of an overgrowth in apparatus-based diagnostics and this is to a not inconsiderable extent responsible for the explosion in costs which we are now experiencing in medicine and which threaten to crush us. If we register that, we will not, I hope, be accused of preaching a return to the "good old days"; and it may be stressed that "this part of the diagnostics is more rapid and certain." Equipment *should* be used, but only following sound indications obtained from a medical examination with accurate anamnesis. But it must be emphasized here that computer tomography and some of "technological" methods have led, owing to false interpretation, even to false diagnoses – because of the absence of data from a clinical preexamination. These could, with a more exact indication, well-documented anamnesis and neurological findings, have been avoided.

Thus we should take with us, as neurologists, one guiding principle from this discussion: we should not forget the "old tools" of the exact neurological examination which will bring us again on to the path of the relationship of close confidence to the patient.

Just where the path leads to at the end of this century we do not know. In the earlier exposition of this theme (1969), some views were expressed which have proved, to a greater or lesser extent, to belong to the realms of imagination. Percival Bailey once said: we neurologists should also be able to dream at some time. Thus, let us dream of a healthier world with measured and controlled advances which we can unequivocally accept. We want then to work for this with all our strength.

I have reached the end of my report and wish you all a stimulating and productive period of time spent at the conference in the city of Hamburg and in that country, whose history, as regards neurology, I have here tried to relate.

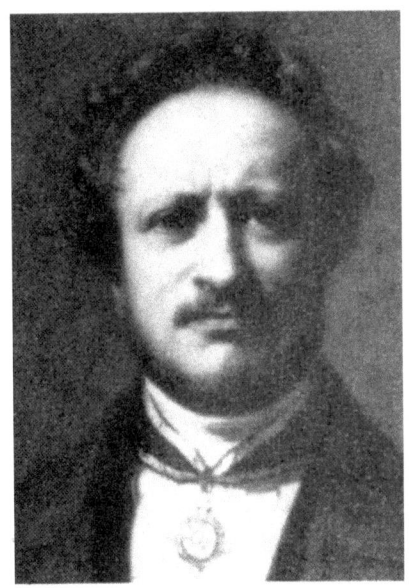

Abb./Fig. 1
Johannes Müller
1801–1858

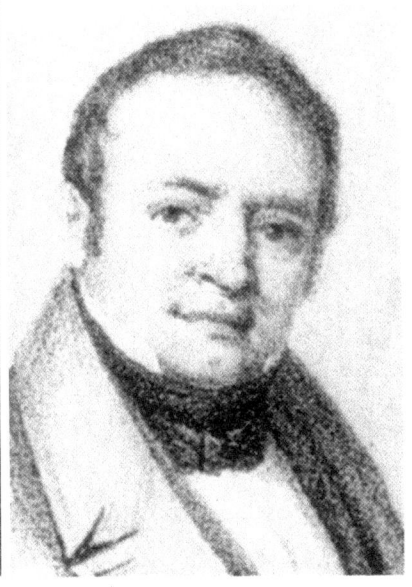

Abb./Fig. 2
Moritz-Heinrich Romberg
1786–1873

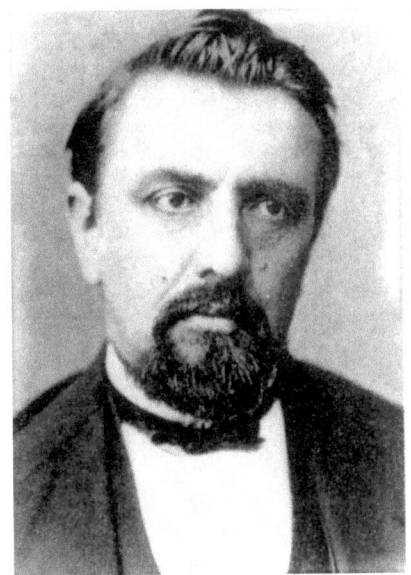

Abb./Fig. 3
Nikolaus Friedreich
1825–1882

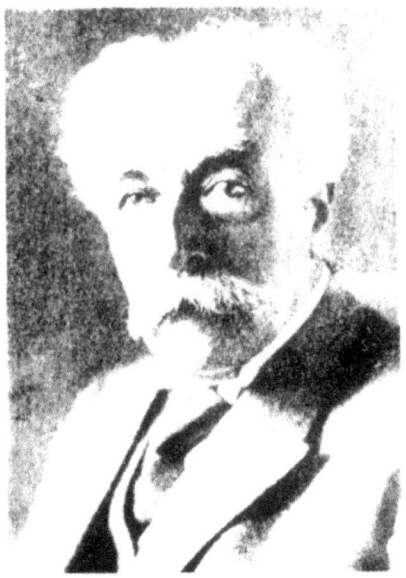

Abb./Fig. 4
Adolf Strümpell
1856–1925

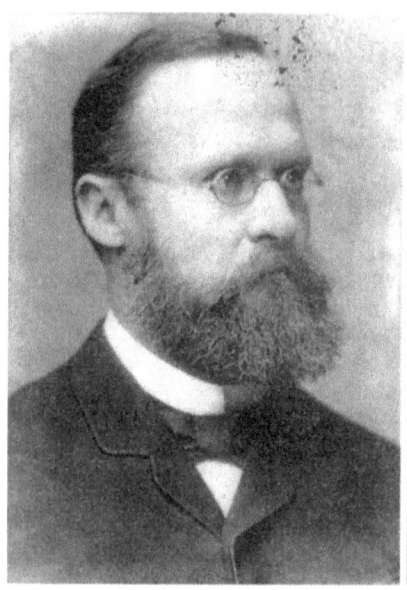

Abb./Fig. 5
Wilhelm Erb
1840–1921

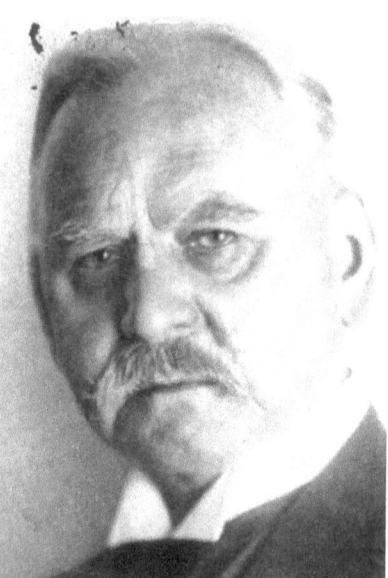

Abb./Fig. 6
Max Nonne
1861–1959

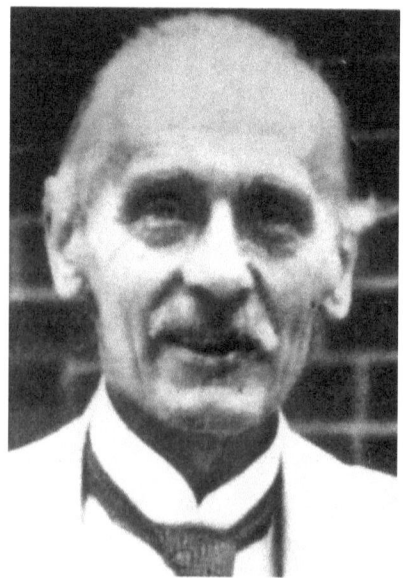

Abb./Fig. 7
Otfrid Foerster
1873–1941

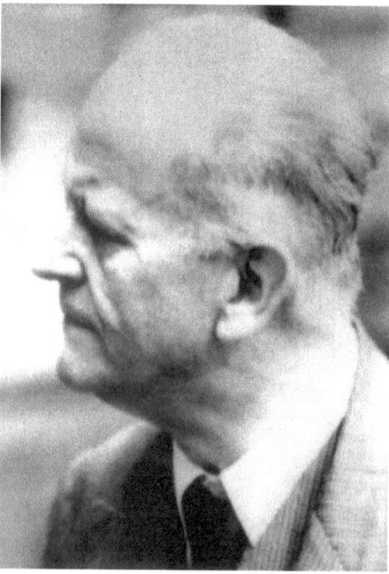

Abb./Fig. 8
Viktor von Weizsäcker
1886–1957

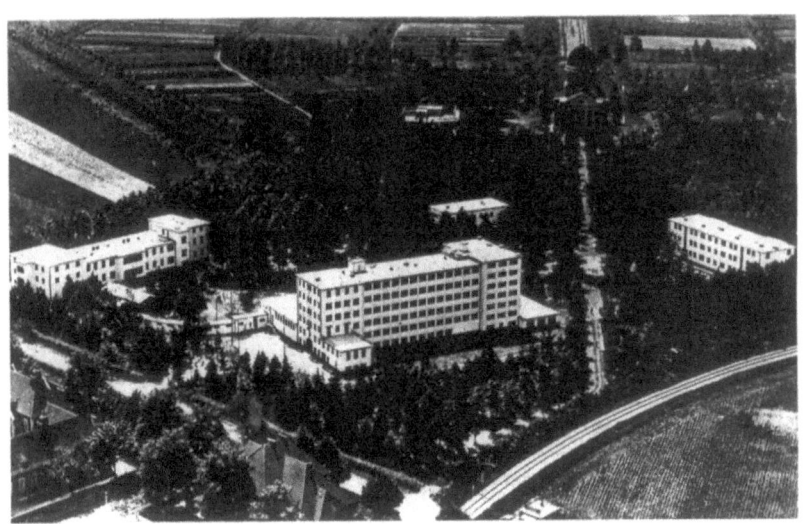

Abb./Fig. 9
Kaiser Wilhelm Institut Berlin-Buch

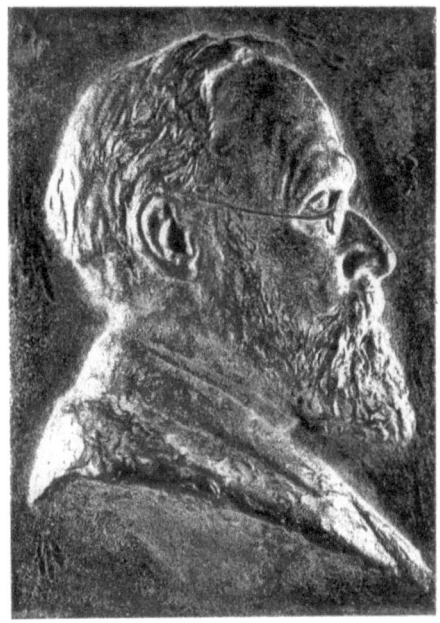

Abb./Fig. 10
Wilhelm Erb Commemoration Medal

Schrifttum – Bibliography

Behrend, R. C., Gänshirt, H., Hallen, O., Janz, D., Kalm, H.: Neurologie und Psychiatrie. Nervenarzt 33, 245–248 (1962).
Zülch, K. J.: Der Stand der Neurologie in der Medizin und ihre Zukunft. Privatdruck des Max-Planck-Institutes für Hirnforschung, Abteilung für allgemeine Neurologie, Köln-Merheim 1963 (dort auch Literatur).
Zülch, K. J.: The place of neurology in medicine and its future. In: Vinken, P. J., Bruyn, B. W. (Eds.): Handbook of Clinical Neurology, vol. 1, North Holland Publ., Amsterdam 1969, 1–44 (dort auch Literatur).
Zülch, K. J.: Die Stellung der Neurologie unter den medizinischen Disziplinen. In: Semper Attentus – Beiträge für Heinz Götze zum 8. August 1977. Springer, Berlin Heidelberg New York 1977, 341–354.
Zülch, K. J.: Development of Neurology. In: Wolman, B. B. (Ed.): Encyclopedia of Psychiatry, Psychology, Psychoanalysis and Neurology, vol. 5. Van Nostrand Reinhold, New York 1977, 198–201.
Zülch, K. J.: The Present State of Neurology in the World. Neurologia Psichiatria Science Umane 3, 1–24 (1983).
Zutt, J.: Psychiatrie und Neurologie. Nervenarzt 33, 1–6, 275–277 (1962); 35, 175–176 (1964).
Zutt, J.: Das Frankfurter Nervenzentrum. Tagung mit Unterstützung der Dr. Karl Thomae GmbH, Frankfurt 1964.

Genauere Biographien der erwähnten Wissenschaftler:
More detailed biographies of the scientists:

Dumesnil, R.: Schadewaldt, H.: Die berühmten Ärzte. 2. deutsche Auflage. Aulis-Verlag Deubner & Co, Köln 1966.
Haymaker, W., Schiller, F.: The Founders of Neurology. 2nd Edn. Thomas, Springfield/Illinois 1970.
Kolle, K.: Die großen Nervenärzte. Thieme, Stuttgart, Band I 1955, Band II 1959, Band III 1963.

MIX
Papier aus verantwortungsvollen Quellen
Paper from responsible sources
FSC® C105338

If you have any concerns about our products,
you can contact us on
ProductSafety@springernature.com

In case Publisher is established outside the EU,
the EU authorized representative is:
**Springer Nature Customer Service Center GmbH
Europaplatz 3, 69115 Heidelberg, Germany**

Printed by Libri Plureos GmbH
in Hamburg, Germany